WHY WON'T SOMEONE HELP ME?

GLADYS QUINTAL

ISBN: 149364114X
ISBN-13: 978-1493641147

DEDICATION

To my GP, my new integrated thyroid doctor, my chiropractor, my endocrine surgeon and all of the supportive friends I have made along the way – thank you so much for believing in me and giving me my life back.

CONTENTS

Chapter 1

I must admit that in my early 20's I wasn't exactly empathetic to other people's ailments. They would complain of flu's or bad backs – things I had never experienced and so compassion wasn't exactly flowing out of me. Karma was about to bite me on the bum, big time.

I had always been relatively healthy; healthy weight, good blood pressure, slept pretty well, ate healthily and exercised regularly. The first time I woke up with pain in my lower back at the age of 23, I thought I was dying! I went to see the local chiropractor who did a few manipulations and told me I needed to take care; not to use my back like a crane, bend my knees etc. I thought that was the end of it. I got a few niggles now and again and needed cataflam or voltarin, but mostly it was fine.

Then one day at age 29, I thought I had my very first bout of flu. I hurt everywhere. Every muscle ached, I was bedridden and had no idea what was going on. I didn't seem to have a temperature, sore throat or sniffles – but I felt as if I had been hit by a bus. The next day however, I was fine. A miraculous recovery, so it couldn't have been influenza.

Not long after this 'flu' episode the fatigue hit me, pretty much out of the blue. I found myself getting tired really easily and went to my doctor to get it checked out. He took it pretty seriously as the only times I went to him normally were for contraception, my pregnancies or my children were sick. He sent me for x-rays of my back which was giving me a bit of grief now and did a bunch of blood tests. He also started giving me weekly vitamin B12 injections. Nothing of significance showed in my blood, but he said I had the spine of an old lady and really needed to take care of it from now on.

Things started to go downhill from there. I found I couldn't walk as far as I used to, my shins would hurt. My right shoulder would ache when I was hanging out the washing and the fatigue was getting harder and harder to deal with. I had no idea what was going on, but thought it must be some type of arthritis. I took anti – inflammatories for the pain and just tried to get through each day. I was working 30hrs a week and had my daughter to get to and from school each day. I was coping, just.

I suddenly started to get reflux, acid indigestion and it was not just after eating something spicy – it was all the time. The doctor sent me off for a gastroscopy to check nothing sinister was going on. I was diagnosed with G.O.R.D and put on Losec. This helped but he also noticed that my blood pressure seemed to be creeping up. I started to have heart palpitations and chest tightness and ended up on bp meds soon after. At this stage I was starting to get a tad depressed with all these different ailments and medications going on and then the weight started to pile on! Talk about kicking you while you are down....

I found it hard to exercise much anymore, I was craving sugar and starchy food all the time and the fatigue was getting worse and worse. During all this upheaval, we had been trying to get pregnant as my age was creeping up quickly and I was scared I would be too old if I waited until I was well again – if I ever got well again.

Chapter 2

Four miscarriages and a lot of heartache later, we were almost at the point of giving up. Doctors couldn't find any reason why this was happening – I had 2 healthy children already but for some reason now I was having fertility problems. We had genetic tests and ultrasounds and every blood test under the sun. I decided to go off all the pregnancy vitamins and forget about a baby for a while. Then I got pregnant again and this time I carried til term. My bp behaved itself until around 34 weeks and I had gestational diabetes towards the end. Our baby boy was born with low blood sugar and jaundice and had to spend a few days in the neo-natal unit. My bp was going haywire post delivery and they were having trouble controlling it. Two weeks after his birth, we were finally allowed to go home. I had fed my daughter for almost a year and didn't envisage any problems this time. But after torturing myself for months with a baby not gaining weight properly and a stressed out mother and father, I put him on the bottle and he settled immediately. I felt like a failure and wondered why it was so hard this time.

I began to wonder if somehow the vitamins had something to do with the miscarriages? It was the only thing I had done differently and I hadn't taken them with the two older kids. I tried desperately to lose weight and improve my health, but it seemed to slowly deteriorate. I was still pretty active, but I was tired a lot. Hubby put it down to age and having a baby at 39, but I just knew there was more to it.

When our son was around 18months we made the decision to move from NZ to Western Australia. I was very excited to start our new life and went about joining playgroups and creating a new circle of friends. We did a lot and were very social and a little while later started to think about having another baby. My GP thought it would be a good idea to get checked out as I was 41 now. All tests came back normal. I had lost about 14kg and on the surface seemed healthy enough. The only problem found was a gallbladder filled to the brim with stones and it was recommended that I have this removed before thinking about becoming pregnant – which I did.

We stopped using contraception and thought we would just see what happened. We knew after all the prior problems we had been extremely fortunate to have a baby and so decided not to put any pressure on ourselves and just count ourselves lucky. If it happened it happened. But it didn't – nothing happened. So we just forgot about another baby and got on with our lives. My health took a turn for the worse and I started to gain weight and feel really bad again. I sat down one day and wrote a list of all my symptoms, including: weight gain, fatigue, all over muscle pain, brain fog, reflux, high blood pressure, heart palpitations, constipation, weakness and dizziness. I took the list into my GP and asked if there was any way they could all be connected. He looked at me and said he doubted it, but if they were I probably didn't want to know about it. He suggested because of my age and fertility problems it could be peri-menopause. He did a bunch of blood tests and referred me to a neurologist and cardiologist.

The neurologist suspected MS, though he thought it was unlikely. He booked me in for an MRI and did blood tests – everything came back clear and so he suggested I look at anti anxiety drugs. I took offense to this, as I knew it was more than just being anxious. The illness was making me anxious – not the other way around.

The cardiologist referred me for a heart scan, monitor and stress test. All came back normal except for an irregular heartbeat. They suggested getting my thyroid checked. The GP had already done thyroid tests that were all normal and so I was once again considered a mystery.

Chapter 3

We bought a house and I started to think about going back to work in the next year or so when our son would be at school. Then both my feet suddenly swelled up. My GP sent me to a rheumatologist who promptly diagnosed me with Fibromyalgia. At last I had a diagnosis! She prescribed me a low dose anti depressant to help me sleep and medications for the pain. There was no cure, but at least I knew I wasn't going crazy. I resigned myself to the fact that this was my lot in life and tried to get on with it as best I could.

I realised that the sun seemed to make my symptoms worse and so tried to avoid it as much as possible – which is no easy feat living in Western Australia! I could no longer run around with my son and was slowly retreating to the sidelines to watch the fun instead of joining in. It was very hard and I felt cheated, but there was nothing I could do about it.

We decided to buy a bigger house, ours was a very small three bedroom and we didn't have a spare room or any storage. We bought a house close to the school and a few months later, at the age of 45, I discovered I was pregnant. To say it was a shock was an understatement. I expected to miscarry and was walking on eggshells most of the time. I started bleeding at 21 weeks but the baby was fine, thank God. Although it was a pregnancy plagued with health issues: pre-eclampsia, cholestasis, gestational diabetes (I was injecting myself with insulin 4 times a day) and of course the pre-existing fibro – I was induced at 38 weeks and had a very healthy baby girl weighing 7lb 7oz.

I had the same feeding issues again and after persevering for a while, gave in and put her on the bottle and she thrived. She was such a blessing and I couldn't believe that at 45 with all my health and weight issues, I could be so incredibly lucky.

Then when our baby was around 9months old, my bp shot up suddenly – dangerously high and wouldn't come down. I was home alone at the time with a 6year old and a baby and was scared about what to do. I felt as if I was going to pass out. I rang my daughter who was 19 and living with her boyfriend now and asked her to come and watch the kids so I could go to the doctor. Then stupidly drove myself there!

The after-hours surgery was packed and I was worried I was going to faint right there on the floor. I told the receptionist that I was fighting to stay conscious and if possible could I see the doctor urgently. She said I looked like all the blood had drained out of my face and took me straight in. Next thing I know, I am getting loaded into an ambulance, trying to organise someone to pick up my car and getting my daughter to stay the night with my babies. Hubby was beside himself as he couldn't get home that night. It was a horrible situation, something I wouldn't wish on anyone.

I was terrified I was going to die. I had 4 kids, including a beautiful baby that needed me – I needed to get through this. While giving my history to the doctors at the ER (Fibromyalgia, hypertension, irregular heartbeat etc) one doctor seemed very interested in my case. He asked me if I had been checked for an adrenal tumour, had my thyroid checked etc. He ran a few blood tests and arranged for me to see a cardiologist again.

I was monitored for 2 nights and declared fine to go home – noting on my discharge papers that I had a high calcium reading.

Chapter 4

What the hell did high calcium mean? I had never heard of it before, always seen the Caltrate adds talking about osteo and low calcium, but never high calcium. As soon as I got home and had a spare second, I googled it. Googling high calcium took me directly to parathyroid.com and I was to have a new education.

Not only had I never heard of high calcium, but I had never heard of a parathyroid gland either. Four little glands, about the size of a grain of rice, positioned behind your thyroid – their sole purpose: controlling the amount of calcium circulating in your blood. I was to learn about a disease called hyperparathyroidism, where one or more of these glands grows and becomes hyper, stripping calcium from your bones and putting it into your bloodstream.

Symptoms included: Fatigue, weight gain, reflux, mood swings, brain fog, bone pain, constipation, depression – hang on a minute, this was me! I had all these symptoms and had the high calcium to boot. I had hyperparathyroidism and according to this site it could be cured by a simple operation. Cured? I could be cured? This was a miracle and now all I needed to do was to get the doctor to refer me for surgery. Or so I thought…..

Diagnosing myself via Dr Google was one thing, but finding a real life doctor to back up that diagnosis was something else. I took the reports from the hospital along to my GP and asked for further testing. He ordered a PTH blood test along with vitamin D, referred me for a sestamibi radioactive scan and referred me to an endocrinologist. All the right things to do.

The PTH test came back high – way above normal but the vitamin D was very, very low. I had read on the internet that this was common with HPT. The body's own defence mechanism – lower the vitamin D to stop the body absorbing any more calcium. It made perfect sense to me and yet all the doctors saw was 'low vitamin D' and decided that this was my problem.

The first endocrinologist I saw had made her mind up before even setting eyes on me! She was extremely rude and condescending, telling me that my problem was low vitamin D causing secondary HPT and that all I needed was supplements and my parathyroids would settle down, physio and acupuncture would help with the pain. I had visions of just where I would like the acupuncturist to put those needles! She also said that my pain was in no way connected to my high calcium and didn't want to explain to me how my calcium was high if my D was so low.

I went home feeling a little depressed but glad that I already had an appointment for the scan. Hoping it would show something and prove her wrong. How could she treat me like that – she didn't even know me?

I went home and went online again to research the vitamin D/secondary HPT thing. Most sites said it was caused by kidney failure, though a few believed low levels of vitamin D were the cause of parathyroid glands going hyper. The only problem with her secondary theory was that the calcium never went high.

I joined a few pages on Facebook about HPT and met a lot of people in the same position. I learnt just how hard it was to get properly diagnosed and to get surgery. I found out that a lot of suffers also had low thyroid function and that when doctors ordered thyroid tests, they only ordered the TSH (Thyroid Stimulating Hormone) and not the actual thyroid hormones at all. Sestamibi scans could be a good location tool, but weren't a diagnostic tool. Blood and symptoms were used to diagnose. I made some really good friends on those sites and talked to a few who had surgery and were cured. Some had needed second surgeries and some had surgery but their adenomas were never found. I hoped that wasn't going to be me, I desperately needed to be cured.

I went back to my GP and asked for the thyroid tests to be done. I asked for TSH, FT3, FT4 and antibodies and though albeit reluctantly, he obliged. I was so sure those tests were going to come back abnormal and that together with getting my surgery, I would get my thyroid sorted and be on the way back to health.

I went back a week later. He had already printed my results out and practically threw them at me before I had even the chance to sit down.

"Your thyroid is fine, you don't need drugs," he snapped at me.

I felt terrible, like a fraud and left with my tail between my legs. Drugs? Why did he say it like that? I had an aversion to drugs and hardly took any pain meds. Did he think I was only after drugs?

Chapter 5

I had my scan, which took a lot out of me. Lying still for 30-40 mins at a time was really hard on my back. But I did it and then prayed that my adenoma would glow like a light bulb and prove to everyone that I wasn't crazy. The scan came back inconclusive, but my entire right thyroid lobe had a way stronger uptake than the left. This told me that the adenoma was there, behind that lobe or embedded in it.

After speaking to one girl quite a bit in South Australia, we became quite close. She told me a lot about how to read tests etc and about the ranges. I joined a few thyroid sites under her advice and learnt that my thyroid wasn't fine, it was just scraping inside the range and I was hypothyroid. She was corresponding with a surgeon in Sydney and managed to get him to agree to operate. She flew over by herself for the surgery, spent a few days in a motel alone after surgery and then flew back alone. So brave she was and it terrified the hell out of me! I wanted surgery so desperately – was I going to have to travel as well?

I got her surgeon's email address from her and wrote to him, telling him my story and asking who he would recommend in WA. He recommended a good endocrine surgeon, wished me luck and asked to keep him informed. He was very nice – totally different to the endo I had seen recently.

Armed with this new information, I went back to a different GP and asked to be referred directly to this surgeon. He was reluctant as he was convinced I was suffering from depression and needed injections of vitamin D to bring it up faster. No way did I want that! The pills I was already taking made me feel terrible and I didn't want to risk having a stroke if the D caused my calcium to go sky high. He reluctantly agreed to the referral, but wanted to talk therapy and physio on our next visit. I also managed to get a thyroid ultrasound referral – telling a little white lie, that the surgeon has requested I get one done before the appointment.

I had the ultrasound which showed my right lobe to be slightly enlarged and that I had 2 cysts. I was more convinced than ever that the right side was where it was at and needed to get the surgeon to agree.

I had more bloods done, my PTH was all over the place. Four times it was high, a couple of times normal and my calcium was mostly high/normal. For my PTH to be high and calcium high/normal – again this was proof to me that I had an enlarged gland. They are meant to be at opposite ends of the scale if my parathyroids were working as they should be. If PTH is high, calcium should be on the low side and vice versa. But the low vitamin D was confusing everyone and at this stage it was still just under normal on the scale.

The surgeon was lovely, he agreed there was a hot spot on the sestamibi and that my PTH was high and calcium high/normal – out of range high once as well. He did a metabolic bone study that came back normal and so that was no help to me. But the low D complicated things even more for him and he wanted me to get a second opinion and see another endocrinologist. I let him refer me even though I knew what to expect already. I upped my vitamin D in the hopes of getting my levels up and ended up bedridden for 2days. How on earth was I going to get this surgery? The appointment to see the second endo seemed to take forever and in the meantime I was going downhill fast.

Chapter 6

I found it really hard to drive long distances now and the appointment was about an hour away. My hubby drove me there and watched our baby while I went in alone – I wish to God he had come in with me now or that I had recorded our conversation, because I don't think he honestly believes it was as bad as I say it was. Truth be told, it was probably worse!

At first he seemed really nice, but I think maybe that was a front to give me a false sense of security so he could get me totally off guard while he went in for the kill. He asked me some questions about my symptoms, family history, home life etc and then gave me his opinion. As far as he was concerned there was absolutely nothing wrong with me that high doses of vitamin D, antidepressants and anti-inflammatories couldn't fix. If I didn't stop my naughtiness and take my medications – his actual words – there was nothing anyone could do to help me. I needed my husband home more as I was pining for him....what am I, 16?

I tried to tell him how the D made me feel and he said that was rubbish, it was probably the fact I wasn't taking enough. I said how the anti-inflams interfered with my bp meds. He asked who told me that? The chemist, ambulance officer, cardiologist....once again this was just rubbish and I was just clutching at straws and making up excuses.

I left his office not sad, but very angry. How dare he speak to me like that? I came to the conclusion that once he sent his report to my surgeon, I could kiss any hopes of an operation goodbye. I decided to try another surgeon in WA – but he thought along the same lines. Was this the way it was? Unless my calcium and PTH went sky high and my D was normal – I was going to be left to suffer.

I was feeling pretty depressed and desperate now. No one really understood – I looked fine on the outside. I was grossly overweight by now and am pretty sure a lot of people thought that was my main problem, even hubby unfortunately. I knew I had to lose weight, but it was impossible feeling like this and the fatigue was so debilitating. I could take pain meds but nothing helped with that fatigue. It was like someone was slipping sedatives into my coffee or something and I was struggling to push through it every day.

Towards the end, I was needing Nana naps every day and felt as though I just wasn't getting any sleep at all. I was scared to drive too far for fear of falling asleep. I would have to take my daughter with me to make sure I remembered where I was going. I did have a couple of really good friends that did understand and of course my forum friends that helped to keep me sane and believing it was not all in my head. Thank goodness I had enough sense to have a support group behind me!

Chapter 7

I had another episode one night with a bp spike and ended up in hospital again. This time they checked my parathyroid hormone and calcium which were both high. Vitamin D was now normal. I started to get really down and seemed to see no light at the end of the tunnel. Hubby asked me why I was taking the vitamin D if it made me feel so bad – I told him I had needed to get the level up if there was any hope of getting surgery and now that it was normal, I would stop taking it.

I thought about a plan B and researched other surgeons out of state. My friend had heard of a lovely surgeon over east that had helped a few people and so I made the decision to email her. She was very nice and agreed with me that I probably did have an adenoma. She said she would consider surgery if I was prepared to treat it as another diagnostic tool. Meaning if she went in and found nothing, I could live with that and move on. Since I didn't have insurance and I couldn't be put on the public waiting list outside of state – my only option was to pay for surgery myself.

I didn't think hubby would even consider this option, pay thousands of dollars for me to fly to the other side of Australia for a surgery he wasn't even convinced would help me. But he did, he even suggested it before I had the chance to mention it to him. We refinanced the house and got the money together and then a little voice in the back of my head told me to try the surgeon here just once more – what could it hurt?

So, I wrote him this big long letter. I told him that my vitamin D was now in the normal range, my last PTH and calcium were both high and that I was not a poor, pathetic housewife as the endocrinologist had implied.

I also reminded him of the hotspot on the sestamibi and that I believed I either had an enlarged gland behind the right lobe or embedded in it. I also told him how I planned to go out of state for surgery, but had decided just one last time to try and get surgery locally.

It worked! I couldn't believe it. He wrote back and told me to make an appointment with his secretary and to bring everything with me; scans, blood tests etc. He looked at everything and then booked me in for surgery for 3 weeks time. I must have looked like an idiot – I couldn't wipe the smile off my face! His secretary gave me the forms to fill in and a number to ring the hospital and book a pre-assessment interview, which I did.

A few days before surgery was due, I got a phone call from the nurse doing the assessment. She said she didn't mean to sound rude, but had I put my height and weight down right? I had gallbladder surgery there 4 years ago and seemed to have gained a lot of weight since then. Of course I had put it down right, which meant that I didn't meet the BMI criteria for surgery at the hospital. Sorry, but no surgery for you.

To say I was devastated would be the understatement of the century – I was lost, what did I do now? I had tried losing weight, gone to both Jenny Craig and Sureslim and both had ended up telling me I had a medical reason hindering weight loss, most likely my thyroid. What was I meant to do now?

I rang the surgeon and got his secretary. He was out of the office today, but she would consult with him and get back to me. I felt like such a loser, too fat for surgery. It was embarrassing and a vicious cycle. I couldn't lose weight without surgery and I couldn't have surgery unless I lost weight. The wait to hear back was horrible.

She rang back a few hours later after talking to him. She said he had been shocked and that he didn't think I was that big. He had suggested that I rebook at a different hospital and go from there. She booked me into another hospital in a few weeks time and all was well with the world again.

Chapter 8

I can't tell you just how nervous I was leading up to surgery. I know, I know – I had practically begged to have this operation, but the thing that scared me the most was the anticipation of being wheeled into theatre and put to sleep. That was the part that terrified me, not the actual surgery!

I had been through so many GP's at this stage, just not happy with the care I had received. I had a couple of really, really good ones – but they had left the area and abandoned me. I kind of felt as if it was me against the world, although I did feel as if my surgeon was now in my corner too. That was a nice feeling, someone willing to take a chance on me.

All the stress of the upcoming surgery as well as impending trip to NZ (a whole other story!) was taking its toll on me and my blood pressure was all over the place. It was erratic and I was having heart palpitations. Now I was worried that this could postpone my surgery once again. I rang the medical centre and made an appointment to see any doctor that was free. It turned out to be the new guy that had just started a few days ago.

I had to fill him in on my history and the fast approaching surgery and ask for help to get my bp down in time for the surgery in just over a week. He seemed very concerned that my blood pressure was so high and asked a lot of questions. He examined me, tested reflexes, listened to my chest etc and then took his stethoscope out of his ears, looked at me and proclaimed that I was Hypothyroid.

Then I – like the strong willed and independent woman I was – proceeded to burst into tears and make a complete dick of myself! I had just not expected it. I had been telling doctors for years that my thyroid function was low, that I needed it tested – not just the TSH but all the thyroid hormones and antibodies. Here was this doctor that had never laid eyes on me before today, telling me this without me even having to mention it.

He helped me down off the bed and over to a chair. He told me it was ok, he could see I had been dealing with this a long time and had been trying to be strong – but now we would sort it out. It would all be ok. He said there wasn't much point in doing the thyroid tests now this close to surgery, but at the 6-8week mark post surgery, we would do tests and see where my thyroid was at.

I felt as if someone had just reached down from the heavens and taken a huge weight off my shoulders. He upped my bp meds and told me to come back in a few days. It took a lot to get it back down and the night before surgery I took anti anxiety meds to help keep me calm.

Hubby decided that since the hospital was so far away and I had to be at there at 6am, we should all go the day before and stay the night down there. We booked a lovely 2 bedroom cabin at a local holiday park a few minutes' drive from the hospital and everything was set.

Although I had been terrified leading up to surgery, strangely on the day I was very calm. They took me to the hospital, waited a little while and then left. My obs were done – blood pressure was very good – and I was put in a room in the queue for surgery. I hadn't eaten or drank anything from midnight but I wasn't hungry at all, just anxious to get it over with. I wasn't scared of the surgery as such, just the anaesthetic. I knew from experience how bad I felt afterwards from it. Nausea, chest pain and just totally wiped out. Plus that waiting for the anaesthetic to be put in was not a favourite pastime of mine.

I was soon to figure out that I was last in line for surgery for that day. Before I knew it, it was lunchtime and I was still waiting. At 3pm an orderly finally arrived to take me to theatre. I had been at the hospital waiting for 9hours. I felt a little nervous, but just kept telling myself that it would all be over soon. He wheeled me into the little alcove and a nurse came over straight away and checked everything was right. Then the anaesthetist came over. I double checked that he knew my BMI – it was really playing on my mind now. At that point my surgeon came over. I told him I thought he had forgotten me and he smiled. Then I said that maybe he was hoping by starving me all day, my BMI might be lower. The anaesthetist grabbed my hand and said. "Honey, you are not even my second biggest patient for the day – you don't phase me."

I had to laugh and next thing I knew, I was being wheeled into theatre. So different to the experiences I had previously, not scary at all.

Once in there, the anaesthetist starts hitting the back of my hand really hard. He was trying to find a vein – unsuccessfully since I hadn't had anything to drink for about 21 hours! He put a needle in and it didn't work.

"Oh great," I said. "Don't tell me you are going to have to do it again?"

"We can do it without anaesthetic if you like?" he said, looking almost excited.

I was laughing so much I couldn't believe I was in an operating theatre.

Then behind me I heard my surgeon's voice.

"Which side was the hotspot on again?"

"Great," I said, "feeling really confident here!"

I hadn't even noticed that the anaesthetist had put the cannula into my vein.

"He is just pulling your leg. Going to give you a little something now," he said, emptying a syringe into my arm.

Chapter 9

I woke up in recovery with terrible chest pains and nausea. There were doctors and nurses all around me, taking my blood pressure and asking me questions. They gave me anti-nausea meds and meds in case I was having a heart attack and took me back to my room.

They wanted to take me for a chest x-ray but the surgeon had left strict instructions that I was to be propped up and the nurse said they would have to bring the portable x-ray machine in and so they did. My back was killing me, someone gave me tramadol which I promptly threw up. My heart rate was erratic and this really worried them, they kept doing ECG's. I told them that irregular was normal for me, but they still kept a very close eye on me.

The night nurse made me a heat pack for my back that practically eased the pain instantly – so simple and yet so effective. I had no pain in my throat at all and once the nausea and chest pain subsided, it wasn't too bad at all. I managed to get a little sleep and was up and down to the toilet a few times.

The surgeon came in the next day and told me he had removed one enlarged parathyroid gland and my entire right thyroid lobe. He had checked the other parathyroids – but had only found 3, number 4 was elusive. I secretly hoped number 4 was normal.

I was fine to go home and was to see him again in 2 weeks.

So I went home. I was lucky that I had my Facebook HPT friends to tell me what to expect so I was ok when my heart started racing or I got cramps or pins and needles. The thyroid can go a little hyper following surgery, causing anxiety, racing heart, night sweats etc and it can take a while for the healthy parathyroids to wake up and start regulating calcium properly again. Low calcium symptoms are cramps, tingles or shaking – sometimes headaches and anxiety too. Thanks to my support group friends, I was prepared.

I really noticed the change within days. I was tired after surgery and the anaesthetic always knocks me around a bit, but I still felt way better than I did before the operation. I noticed I could sit out in the sun and not feel terrible afterwards. The fatigue got less and less and my right eye that had been twitching pretty much 24/7 had stopped. I still had the body aches and the reflux and my bp was all over the place – but I felt as if whatever had been slowly poisoning me to death was gone.

As time has gone on, I have gotten better and better. I can now go out with my family and actually join in – instead of watching on the sidelines. I can go shopping and drive if I have to. I am not needing a nap every day and am waking up in the morning actually feeling as if I have been to sleep. I still have the reflux and the muscle pain though. The doctor thinks it may be thyroid related and did the blood tests last week.

I got the blood test results today and I am indeed Hypothyroid as he said and I always knew I was. I am anaemic as well, so I will begin treatment for them soon – it could take a while to get right, but now I know I can fight and get the treatment I deserve. Plus I have a good doctor in my corner now as well. My corner is getting bigger – not just lonely old me anymore.

I wonder if it was the extra calcium in the pregnancy vitamins that caused the miscarriages or the fact that my thyroid function was low. I guess I will never know. I never take anything at face value anymore and if I don't understand anything or disagree with something, then it is Dr Google to the rescue or my friends that have been through it and understand first hand.

The moral of this story? If you think there is something wrong, there probably is – trust your instincts. If you are not happy with the care you are receiving from your doctor, then find another doctor and another and another…. Until you are satisfied he or she has your best interests at heart. Don't just aimlessly take vitamins or supplements without first getting tested to see if you actually are deficient in anything….

It is your life, you shouldn't have to settle if your ailments can be cured and you deserve to live life to the fullest!

A note from the author

My 14year old cat started to drastically drop weight, pant, drink heaps and meow all the time. I took her to the vet and he suspected her thyroid. Blood tests for T4 immediately – diagnosed and on meds within 2days! She is doing so much better and I can't help feeling a tad jealous of my cat – wouldn't it be wonderful if we as humans were treated half as well as our pets?

I found out recently that I have Ankylosing Spontilitis and Helicobacter Pylori. Antibiotics should sort out the H.P. and hopefully cure my reflux. AS is in my family and so came as no big surprise. I am still anaemic, have insulin resistance, high cholesterol, borderline adrenal fatigue and low vitamin D – still. All these things go hand in hand with autoimmune disorders, so you need to address everything – not just thyroid meds or an operation to remove a rogue para.

I am improving day by day and all these things are slowly getting sorted out. One day soon, in the not too distant future, I am praying that I will be close to being my old self again. Fingers crossed!

***

A survivor of sexual abuse, I have recently written the true account of my childhood, titled: Life After Hell: Surviving Sexual Abuse. I have tried to convey what happened to me as well as my journey to finally getting justice.

A lot of my real life experiences have gone into my fictional works, especially The Man of My Dreams where I created a vigilante vampire who kills rapists and child molesters.....

I've loved Vampires and the paranormal ever since I can remember and always envisaged myself writing a book or two on the subject! I have written 4 books in The Dream Series so far: The Man of my Dreams, Be Careful What You Wish For, The Chosen One and the 4th book in the series: Succubus: An Erotic Companion which is due for release December 1st. All Paranormal Romance novels with Vampires (of course) as well as a bit of blood and gore thrown in and the 4th one is slightly on the erotic side!

http://thedreamseries-gladysquintal.blogspot.com

Made in the USA
San Bernardino, CA
11 October 2014